The Beauty Entrepreneur

WEEKLY PLANNER

www. deborahlmccampbell.com

Slaying All Day!

MONDAY

WEEKEND

TUESDAY

Goals
FOR THE WEEK

WEDNESDAY

THURSDAY

TO DO:

Task	Done
	☐
	☐
	☐
	☐
	☐
	☐
	☐
	☐

FRIDAY

This Week's Affirmation:

Set goals and slay them.

Weekly Average Ticket Tracker

Knowing your average ticket tells you what each client is spending for their services and retail products.

Step1: Enter Your Info

Line 1: Total Service Dollar $_____
(enter the weekly amt. client spent only)

Line 2: Total Retail Dollars $_____
(enter the weekly amt. client spent only)

Line 3: Total # of Clients. _____
(enter the total amt. of clients serviced per week)

Step 2: Calculate The Information:

Line 4: Your Average Ticket. $_____
(take line 1 total service dollars and divide by the total # of clients from line 3).

Line 5: Your Average Retail Ticket $_____
(take line 2 your total retail dollars and divide by the total # of clients from line 3).

Base Price Budget Worksheet

Knowing your base price calculation will help you to structure your prices for your business and tells you what you need to charge each client in order to stay in business.

Follow the steps below to find out what is your Base Price Budget.

Step 1: Enter your information:

Line 1. Total Monthly Expense. $_____
*(enter all your **total monthly expenses**)*

Line 2. Projected Monthly Profit. $_____
*(enter the amount of profit **you want to make** Each month).*

Line 3. Total # Monthly Client Visits.   _____
*(take the # of services you have, multiply by the # of clients **each person can serve in a month**. You can use your actual client count).*

Step 2: Now calculate the information below:

Line 4: Total projected gross sales $_____
*(take the **total monthly expenses** (line 1) and Add to the **projected monthly profit** (line 2).*

Line 5: Recommended base price
(take the total projected gross sales (line 4) $_____
*And divide the total # **monthly clients visits** (line 3).*

Notes

Slaying All Day!

DATE

__ / __ / __

MONDAY

WEEKEND

TUESDAY

Goals
FOR THE WEEK

WEDNESDAY

TO DO:

Task	Done
	☐
	☐
	☐
	☐
	☐
	☐
	☐
	☐
	☐
	☐

THURSDAY

FRIDAY

This Week's Affirmation:

Girl, you are a Boss.

Weekly Average Ticket Tracker

Knowing your average ticket tells you what each client is spending for their services and retail products.

Step1: Enter Your Info

Line 1: Total Service Dollar $_____
(enter the weekly amt. client spent only)

Line 2: Total Retail Dollars $_____
(enter the weekly amt. client spent only)

Line 3: Total # of Clients. _____
(enter the total amt. of clients serviced per week)

Step 2: Calculate The Information:

Line 4: Your Average Ticket. $_____
(take line 1 total service dollars and divide by the total # of clients from line 3).

Line 5: Your Average Retail Ticket $_____
(take line 2 your total retail dollars and divide by the total # of clients from line 3).

Base Price Budget Worksheet

Knowing your base price calculation will help you to structure your prices for your business and tells you what you need to charge each client in order to stay in business.

Follow the steps below to find out what is your Base Price Budget.

Step 1: Enter your information:

Line 1. Total Monthly Expense. $_____
*(enter all your **total monthly expenses**)*

Line 2. Projected Monthly Profit. $_____
*(enter the amount of profit **you want to make** Each month).*

Line 3. Total # Monthly Client Visits.   _____
*(take the # of services you have, multiply by the # of clients **each person can serve in a month**. You can use your actual client count).*

Step 2: Now calculate the information below:

Line 4: Total projected gross sales $_____
*(take the **total monthly expenses** (line 1) and Add to the **projected monthly profit** (line 2).*

Line 5: Recommended base price
(take the total projected gross sales (line 4) $_____
*And divide the total # **monthly clients visits** (line 3).*

Notes

Slaying All Day!

DATE

__ / __ / __

MONDAY

TUESDAY

WEDNESDAY

THURSDAY

FRIDAY

WEEKEND

Goals
FOR THE WEEK

TO DO:

Task	Done
	☐
	☐
	☐
	☐
	☐
	☐
	☐
	☐
	☐

This Week's Affirmation:

Start your day like the Boss you are.

Weekly Average Ticket Tracker

Knowing your average ticket tells you what each client is spending for their services and retail products.

Step1: Enter Your Info

Line 1: Total Service Dollar $_____
(enter the weekly amt. client spent only)

Line 2: Total Retail Dollars $_____
(enter the weekly amt. client spent only)

Line 3: Total # of Clients. _____
(enter the total amt. of clients serviced per week)

Step 2: Calculate The Information:

Line 4: Your Average Ticket. $_____
(take line 1 total service dollars and divide by the total # of clients from line 3).

Line 5: Your Average Retail Ticket $_____
(take line 2 your total retail dollars and divide by the total # of clients from line 3).

Base Price Budget Worksheet

Knowing your base price calculation will help you to structure your prices for your business and tells you what you need to charge each client in order to stay in business.

Follow the steps below to find out what is your Base Price Budget.

Step 1: Enter your information:

Line 1. Total Monthly Expense. $_____
*(enter all your **total monthly expenses**)*

Line 2. Projected Monthly Profit. $_____
*(enter the amount of profit **you want to make** Each month).*

Line 3. Total # Monthly Client Visits.   _____
*(take the # of services you have, multiply by the # of clients **each person can serve in a month**. You can use your actual client count).*

Step 2: Now calculate the information below:

Line 4: Total projected gross sales $_____
*(take the **total monthly expenses** (line 1) and Add to the **projected monthly profit** (line 2).*

Line 5: Recommended base price
(take the total projected gross sales (line 4) $_____
*And divide the total # **monthly clients visits** (line 3).*

Notes

Slaying All Day!

MONDAY

WEEKEND

TUESDAY

Goals
FOR THE WEEK

WEDNESDAY

TO DO:

Task   **Done**

- ☐
- ☐
- ☐
- ☐
- ☐
- ☐
- ☐
- ☐
- ☐
- ☐
- ☐
- ☐

THURSDAY

FRIDAY

This Week's Affirmation:

I am determined to keep the faith.

Weekly Average Ticket Tracker

Knowing your average ticket tells you what each client is spending for their services and retail products.

Step1: Enter Your Info

Line 1: Total Service Dollar $_____
(enter the weekly amt. client spent only)

Line 2: Total Retail Dollars $_____
(enter the weekly amt. client spent only)

Line 3: Total # of Clients. _____
(enter the total amt. of clients serviced per week)

Step 2: Calculate The Information:

Line 4: Your Average Ticket. $_____
(take line 1 total service dollars and divide by the total # of clients from line 3).

Line 5: Your Average Retail Ticket $_____
(take line 2 your total retail dollars and divide by the total # of clients from line 3).

Knowing your base price calculation will help you to structure your prices for your business and tells you what you need to charge each client in order to stay in business.

Follow the steps below to find out what is your Base Price Budget.

Step 1: Enter your information:

Line 1. Total Monthly Expense. $_____
*(enter all your **total monthly expenses**)*

Line 2. Projected Monthly Profit. $_____
*(enter the amount of profit **you want to make** Each month).*

Line 3. Total # Monthly Client Visits.   _____
*(take the # of services you have, multiply by the # of clients **each person can serve in a month**. You can use your actual client count).*

Step 2: Now calculate the information below:

Line 4: Total projected gross sales $_____
*(take the **total monthly expenses** (line 1) and Add to the **projected monthly profit** (line 2).*

Line 5: Recommended base price
(take the total projected gross sales (line 4) $_____
*And divide the total # **monthly clients visits** (line 3).*

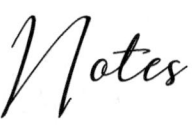

Notes

Slaying All Day!

MONDAY

WEEKEND

TUESDAY

Goals
FOR THE WEEK

WEDNESDAY

TO DO:

Task	Done
	☐
	☐
	☐
	☐

THURSDAY

	☐
	☐
	☐
	☐

FRIDAY

This Week's Affirmation:

Aim higher than yesterday.

Weekly Average Ticket Tracker

Knowing your average ticket tells you what each client is spending for their services and retail products.

Step1: Enter Your Info

Line 1: Total Service Dollar $_____
(enter the weekly amt. client spent only)

Line 2: Total Retail Dollars $_____
(enter the weekly amt. client spent only)

Line 3: Total # of Clients. _____
(enter the total amt. of clients serviced per week)

Step 2: Calculate The Information:

Line 4: Your Average Ticket. $_____
(take line 1 total service dollars and divide by the total # of clients from line 3).

Line 5: Your Average Retail Ticket $_____
(take line 2 your total retail dollars and divide by the total # of clients from line 3).

Base Price Budget Worksheet

Knowing your base price calculation will help you to structure your prices for your business and tells you what you need to charge each client in order to stay in business.

Follow the steps below to find out what is your Base Price Budget.

Step 1: Enter your information:

Line 1. Total Monthly Expense. $_____
(enter all your **total monthly expenses**)

Line 2. Projected Monthly Profit. $_____
(enter the amount of profit **you want to make** Each month).

Line 3. Total # Monthly Client Visits. _____
(take the # of services you have, multiply by the # of clients **each person can serve in a month**. You can use your actual client count).

Step 2: Now calculate the information below:

Line 4: Total projected gross sales $_____
(take the **total monthly expenses** (line 1) and Add to the **projected monthly profit** (line 2).

Line 5: Recommended base price
(take the total projected gross sales (line 4) $_____
And divide the total # **monthly clients visits** (line 3).

Notes

Slaying All Day!

MONDAY

WEEKEND

TUESDAY

Goals
FOR THE WEEK

WEDNESDAY

TO DO:

Task	Done
	☐
	☐
	☐
	☐
	☐
	☐
	☐
	☐
	☐
	☐

THURSDAY

FRIDAY

This Week's Affirmation:

I am more than capable of having a great business.

Weekly Average Ticket Tracker

Knowing your average ticket tells you what each client is spending for their services and retail products.

Step1: Enter Your Info

Line 1: Total Service Dollar $_____
(enter the weekly amt. client spent only)

Line 2: Total Retail Dollars $_____
(enter the weekly amt. client spent only)

Line 3: Total # of Clients. _____
(enter the total amt. of clients serviced per week)

Step 2: Calculate The Information:

Line 4: Your Average Ticket. $_____
(take line 1 total service dollars and divide by the total # of clients from line 3).

Line 5: Your Average Retail Ticket $_____
(take line 2 your total retail dollars and divide by the total # of clients from line 3).

Base Price Budget Worksheet

Knowing your base price calculation will help you to structure your prices for your business and tells you what you need to charge each client in order to stay in business.

Follow the steps below to find out what is your Base Price Budget.

Step 1: Enter your information:

Line 1. Total Monthly Expense. $_____
*(enter all your **total monthly expenses**)*

Line 2. Projected Monthly Profit. $_____
*(enter the amount of profit **you want to make**
Each month).*

Line 3. Total # Monthly Client Visits.   _____
*(take the # of services you have, multiply by the
# of clients **each person can serve in a month**.
You can use your actual client count).*

Step 2: Now calculate the information below:

Line 4: Total projected gross sales $_____
*(take the **total monthly expenses** (line 1) and
Add to the **projected monthly profit** (line 2).*

Line 5: Recommended base price
(take the total projected gross sales (line 4) $_____
*And divide the total # **monthly clients visits**
(line 3).*

Notes

Slaying All Day!

MONDAY

WEEKEND

TUESDAY

Goals FOR THE WEEK

WEDNESDAY

THURSDAY

TO DO:

Task	Done
	☐
	☐
	☐
	☐
	☐
	☐
	☐
	☐
	☐
	☐

FRIDAY

This Week's Affirmation:

The right people will be attracted to me for my business.

Weekly Average Ticket Tracker

Knowing your average ticket tells you what each client is spending for their services and retail products.

Step1: Enter Your Info

Line 1: Total Service Dollar $_____
(enter the weekly amt. client spent only)

Line 2: Total Retail Dollars $_____
(enter the weekly amt. client spent only)

Line 3: Total # of Clients. _____
(enter the total amt. of clients serviced per week)

Step 2: Calculate The Information:

Line 4: Your Average Ticket. $_____
(take line 1 total service dollars and divide by the total # of clients from line 3).

Line 5: Your Average Retail Ticket $_____
(take line 2 your total retail dollars and divide by the total # of clients from line 3).

Base Price Budget Worksheet

Knowing your base price calculation will help you to structure your prices for your business and tells you what you need to charge each client in order to stay in business.

Follow the steps below to find out what is your Base Price Budget.

Step 1: Enter your information:

Line 1. Total Monthly Expense. $_____
*(enter all your **total monthly expenses**)*

Line 2. Projected Monthly Profit. $_____
*(enter the amount of profit **you want to make** Each month).*

Line 3. Total # Monthly Client Visits.   _____
*(take the # of services you have, multiply by the # of clients **each person can serve in a month**. You can use your actual client count).*

Step 2: Now calculate the information below:

Line 4: Total projected gross sales $_____
*(take the **total monthly expenses** (line 1) and Add to the **projected monthly profit** (line 2).*

Line 5: Recommended base price
(take the total projected gross sales (line 4) $_____
*And divide the total # **monthly clients visits** (line 3).*

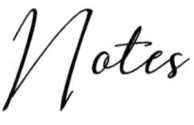

Notes

Slaying All Day!

DATE

__ / __ / __

MONDAY

WEEKEND

TUESDAY

Goals
FOR THE WEEK

WEDNESDAY

TO DO:

Task   **Done**

- [ ]
- [ ]
- [ ]
- [ ]
- [ ]
- [ ]
- [ ]
- [ ]
- [ ]

THURSDAY

FRIDAY

This Week's Affirmation:

Serve with integrity and love and blessings will follow.

Weekly Average Ticket Tracker

Knowing your average ticket tells you what each client is spending for their services and retail products.

Step1: Enter Your Info

Line 1: Total Service Dollar $_____
(enter the weekly amt. client spent only)

Line 2: Total Retail Dollars $_____
(enter the weekly amt. client spent only)

Line 3: Total # of Clients. _____
(enter the total amt. of clients serviced per week)

Step 2: Calculate The Information:

Line 4: Your Average Ticket. $_____
(take line 1 total service dollars and divide by the total # of clients from line 3).

Line 5: Your Average Retail Ticket $_____
(take line 2 your total retail dollars and divide by the total # of clients from line 3).

Base Price Budget Worksheet

Knowing your base price calculation will help you to structure your prices for your business and tells you what you need to charge each client in order to stay in business.

Follow the steps below to find out what is your Base Price Budget.

Step 1: Enter your information:

Line 1. Total Monthly Expense. $_____
*(enter all your **total monthly expenses**)*

Line 2. Projected Monthly Profit. $_____
*(enter the amount of profit **you want to make** Each month).*

Line 3. Total # Monthly Client Visits.   _____
*(take the # of services you have, multiply by the # of clients **each person can serve in a month**. You can use your actual client count).*

Step 2: Now calculate the information below:

Line 4: Total projected gross sales $_____
*(take the **total monthly expenses** (line 1) and Add to the **projected monthly profit** (line 2).*

Line 5: Recommended base price
*(take the total projected gross sales (line 4) $_____ And divide the total # **monthly clients visits** (line 3).*

Notes

Slaying All Day!

DATE

__ __ / __ __ / __ __

MONDAY

WEEKEND

TUESDAY

Goals
FOR THE WEEK

WEDNESDAY

TO DO:

Task   **Done**

☐
☐
☐
☐
☐
☐
☐
☐
☐

THURSDAY

FRIDAY

This Week's Affirmation:

I am bold and fearless to ask for what I want.

Weekly Average Ticket Tracker

Knowing your average ticket tells you what each client is spending for their services and retail products.

Step1: Enter Your Info

Line 1: Total Service Dollar $_____
(enter the weekly amt. client spent only)

Line 2: Total Retail Dollars $_____
(enter the weekly amt. client spent only)

Line 3: Total # of Clients. _____
(enter the total amt. of clients serviced per week)

Step 2: Calculate The Information:

Line 4: Your Average Ticket. $_____
(take line 1 total service dollars and divide by the total # of clients from line 3).

Line 5: Your Average Retail Ticket $_____
(take line 2 your total retail dollars and divide by the total # of clients from line 3).

Base Price Budget Worksheet

Knowing your base price calculation will help you to structure your prices for your business and tells you what you need to charge each client in order to stay in business.

Follow the steps below to find out what is your Base Price Budget.

Step 1: Enter your information:

Line 1. Total Monthly Expense. $_____
*(enter all your **total monthly expenses**)*

Line 2. Projected Monthly Profit. $_____
*(enter the amount of profit **you want to make**
Each month).*

Line 3. Total # Monthly Client Visits.   _____
*(take the # of services you have, multiply by the
# of clients **each person can serve in a month**.
You can use your actual client count).*

Step 2: Now calculate the information below:

Line 4: Total projected gross sales $_____
*(take the **total monthly expenses** (line 1) and
Add to the **projected monthly profit** (line 2).*

Line 5: Recommended base price
(take the total projected gross sales (line 4) $_____
*And divide the total # **monthly clients visits**
(line 3).*

Notes

Slaying All Day!

MONDAY

WEEKEND

TUESDAY

Goals
FOR THE WEEK

WEDNESDAY

TO DO:

Task	Done
	☐
	☐
	☐
	☐
	☐
	☐
	☐
	☐
	☐
	☐

THURSDAY

FRIDAY

This Week's Affirmation:

I am destined to be great.

Weekly Average Ticket Tracker

Knowing your average ticket tells you what each client is spending for their services and retail products.

Step1: Enter Your Info

Line 1: Total Service Dollar $_____
(enter the weekly amt. client spent only)

Line 2: Total Retail Dollars $_____
(enter the weekly amt. client spent only)

Line 3: Total # of Clients. _____
(enter the total amt. of clients serviced per week)

Step 2: Calculate The Information:

Line 4: Your Average Ticket. $_____
(take line 1 total service dollars and divide by the total # of clients from line 3).

Line 5: Your Average Retail Ticket $_____
(take line 2 your total retail dollars and divide by the total # of clients from line 3).

Base Price Budget Worksheet

Knowing your base price calculation will help you to structure your prices for your business and tells you what you need to charge each client in order to stay in business.

Follow the steps below to find out what is your Base Price Budget.

Step 1: Enter your information:

Line 1. Total Monthly Expense. $_____
*(enter all your **total monthly expenses**)*

Line 2. Projected Monthly Profit. $_____
*(enter the amount of profit **you want to make** Each month).*

Line 3. Total # Monthly Client Visits.   _____
*(take the # of services you have, multiply by the # of clients **each person can serve in a month**. You can use your actual client count).*

Step 2: Now calculate the information below:

Line 4: Total projected gross sales $_____
*(take the **total monthly expenses** (line 1) and Add to the **projected monthly profit** (line 2).*

Line 5: Recommended base price
(take the total projected gross sales (line 4) $_____
*And divide the total # **monthly clients visits** (line 3).*

Notes

Slaying All Day!

MONDAY

WEEKEND

TUESDAY

Goals FOR THE WEEK

WEDNESDAY

THURSDAY

TO DO:

Task	Done
	☐
	☐
	☐
	☐
	☐
	☐
	☐
	☐
	☐
	☐

FRIDAY

This Week's Affirmation:

I am attracting positive team members to my business.

Weekly Average Ticket Tracker

Knowing your average ticket tells you what each client is spending for their services and retail products.

Step1: Enter Your Info

Line 1: Total Service Dollar $_____
(enter the weekly amt. client spent only)

Line 2: Total Retail Dollars $_____
(enter the weekly amt. client spent only)

Line 3: Total # of Clients. _____
(enter the total amt. of clients serviced per week)

Step 2: Calculate The Information:

Line 4: Your Average Ticket. $_____
(take line 1 total service dollars and divide by the total # of clients from line 3).

Line 5: Your Average Retail Ticket $_____
(take line 2 your total retail dollars and divide by the total # of clients from line 3).

Base Price Budget Worksheet

Knowing your base price calculation will help you to structure your prices for your business and tells you what you need to charge each client in order to stay in business.

Follow the steps below to find out what is your Base Price Budget.

Step 1: Enter your information:

Line 1. Total Monthly Expense. $_____
*(enter all your **total monthly expenses**)*

Line 2. Projected Monthly Profit. $_____
*(enter the amount of profit **you want to make** Each month).*

Line 3. Total # Monthly Client Visits.   _____
*(take the # of services you have, multiply by the # of clients **each person can serve in a month**. You can use your actual client count).*

Step 2: Now calculate the information below:

Line 4: Total projected gross sales $_____
*(take the **total monthly expenses** (line 1) and Add to the **projected monthly profit** (line 2).*

Line 5: Recommended base price
(take the total projected gross sales (line 4) $_____
*And divide the total # **monthly clients visits** (line 3).*

Notes

Slaying All Day!

DATE

__ / __ / __

MONDAY

TUESDAY

WEDNESDAY

THURSDAY

FRIDAY

WEEKEND

Goals
FOR THE WEEK

TO DO:

Task	Done
	☐
	☐
	☐
	☐
	☐
	☐
	☐
	☐
	☐
	☐

This Week's Affirmation:

Hell yeah, I am building this damn empire.

Weekly Average Ticket Tracker

Knowing your average ticket tells you what each client is spending for their services and retail products.

Step1: Enter Your Info

Line 1: Total Service Dollar $_____
(enter the weekly amt. client spent only)

Line 2: Total Retail Dollars $_____
(enter the weekly amt. client spent only)

Line 3: Total # of Clients. _____
(enter the total amt. of clients serviced per week)

Step 2: Calculate The Information:

Line 4: Your Average Ticket. $_____
(take line 1 total service dollars and divide by the total # of clients from line 3).

Line 5: Your Average Retail Ticket $_____
(take line 2 your total retail dollars and divide by the total # of clients from line 3).

Base Price Budget Worksheet

Knowing your base price calculation will help you to structure your prices for your business and tells you what you need to charge each client in order to stay in business.

Follow the steps below to find out what is your Base Price Budget.

Step 1: Enter your information:

Line 1. Total Monthly Expense. $_____
*(enter all your **total monthly expenses**)*

Line 2. Projected Monthly Profit. $_____
*(enter the amount of profit **you want to make** Each month).*

Line 3. Total # Monthly Client Visits.   _____
*(take the # of services you have, multiply by the # of clients **each person can serve in a month**. You can use your actual client count).*

Step 2: Now calculate the information below:

Line 4: Total projected gross sales $_____
*(take the **total monthly expenses** (line 1) and Add to the **projected monthly profit** (line 2).*

Line 5: Recommended base price
(take the total projected gross sales (line 4) $_____
*And divide the total # **monthly clients visits** (line 3).*

Notes

Slaying All Day!

MONDAY

WEEKEND

TUESDAY

Goals
FOR THE WEEK

WEDNESDAY

THURSDAY

TO DO:

Task   **Done**

☐
☐
☐
☐
☐
☐
☐
☐
☐
☐

FRIDAY

This Week's Affirmation:

I will excel to level up.

Weekly Average Ticket Tracker

Knowing your average ticket tells you what each client is spending for their services and retail products.

Step1: Enter Your Info

Line 1: Total Service Dollar $_____
(enter the weekly amt. client spent only)

Line 2: Total Retail Dollars $_____
(enter the weekly amt. client spent only)

Line 3: Total # of Clients. _____
(enter the total amt. of clients serviced per week)

Step 2: Calculate The Information:

Line 4: Your Average Ticket. $_____
(take line 1 total service dollars and divide by the total # of clients from line 3).

Line 5: Your Average Retail Ticket $_____
(take line 2 your total retail dollars and divide by the total # of clients from line 3).

Base Price Budget Worksheet

Knowing your base price calculation will help you to structure your prices for your business and tells you what you need to charge each client in order to stay in business.

Follow the steps below to find out what is your Base Price Budget.

Step 1: Enter your information:

Line 1. Total Monthly Expense. $_____
*(enter all your **total monthly expenses**)*

Line 2. Projected Monthly Profit. $_____
*(enter the amount of profit **you want to make** Each month).*

Line 3. Total # Monthly Client Visits.   _____
*(take the # of services you have, multiply by the # of clients **each person can serve in a month**. You can use your actual client count).*

Step 2: Now calculate the information below:

Line 4: Total projected gross sales $_____
*(take the **total monthly expenses** (line 1) and Add to the **projected monthly profit** (line 2).*

Line 5: Recommended base price
*(take the total projected gross sales (line 4) $_____
And divide the total # **monthly clients visits** (line 3).*

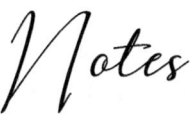

Notes

Slaying All Day!

MONDAY

WEEKEND

TUESDAY

Goals
FOR THE WEEK

WEDNESDAY

TO DO:

Task	Done
	☐
	☐
	☐
	☐
	☐
	☐
	☐
	☐
	☐
	☐

THURSDAY

FRIDAY

This Week's Affirmation:

I am a powerful business woman.

Weekly Average Ticket Tracker

Knowing your average ticket tells you what each client is spending for their services and retail products.

Step1: Enter Your Info

Line 1: Total Service Dollar $_____
(enter the weekly amt. client spent only)

Line 2: Total Retail Dollars $_____
(enter the weekly amt. client spent only)

Line 3: Total # of Clients. _____
(enter the total amt. of clients serviced per week)

Step 2: Calculate The Information:

Line 4: Your Average Ticket. $_____
(take line 1 total service dollars and divide by the total # of clients from line 3).

Line 5: Your Average Retail Ticket $_____
(take line 2 your total retail dollars and divide by the total # of clients from line 3).

Base Price Budget Worksheet

Knowing your base price calculation will help you to structure your prices for your business and tells you what you need to charge each client in order to stay in business.

Follow the steps below to find out what is your Base Price Budget.

Step 1: Enter your information:

Line 1. Total Monthly Expense. $_____
*(enter all your **total monthly expenses**)*

Line 2. Projected Monthly Profit. $_____
*(enter the amount of profit **you want to make** Each month).*

Line 3. Total # Monthly Client Visits.   _____
*(take the # of services you have, multiply by the # of clients **each person can serve in a month**. You can use your actual client count).*

Step 2: Now calculate the information below:

Line 4: Total projected gross sales $_____
*(take the **total monthly expenses** (line 1) and Add to the **projected monthly profit** (line 2).*

Line 5: Recommended base price
(take the total projected gross sales (line 4) $_____
*And divide the total # **monthly clients visits** (line 3).*

Notes

Slaying All Day!

MONDAY

WEEKEND

TUESDAY

Goals
FOR THE WEEK

WEDNESDAY

TO DO:

Task | **Done**

THURSDAY

FRIDAY

This Week's Affirmation:

My business allows me to live the life I have.

Weekly Average Ticket Tracker

Knowing your average ticket tells you what each client is spending for their services and retail products.

Step1: Enter Your Info

Line 1: Total Service Dollar $_____
(enter the weekly amt. client spent only)

Line 2: Total Retail Dollars $_____
(enter the weekly amt. client spent only)

Line 3: Total # of Clients. _____
(enter the total amt. of clients serviced per week)

Step 2: Calculate The Information:

Line 4: Your Average Ticket. $_____
(take line 1 total service dollars and divide by the total # of clients from line 3).

Line 5: Your Average Retail Ticket $_____
(take line 2 your total retail dollars and divide by the total # of clients from line 3).

Base Price Budget Worksheet

Knowing your base price calculation will help you to structure your prices for your business and tells you what you need to charge each client in order to stay in business.

Follow the steps below to find out what is your Base Price Budget.

Step 1: Enter your information:

Line 1. Total Monthly Expense. $_____
*(enter all your **total monthly expenses**)*

Line 2. Projected Monthly Profit. $_____
*(enter the amount of profit **you want to make** Each month).*

Line 3. Total # Monthly Client Visits.   _____
*(take the # of services you have, multiply by the # of clients **each person can serve in a month**. You can use your actual client count).*

Step 2: Now calculate the information below:

Line 4: Total projected gross sales $_____
*(take the **total monthly expenses** (line 1) and Add to the **projected monthly profit** (line 2).*

Line 5: Recommended base price
(take the total projected gross sales (line 4) $_____
*And divide the total # **monthly clients visits** (line 3).*

Notes

Slaying All Day!

MONDAY

WEEKEND

TUESDAY

Goals
FOR THE WEEK

WEDNESDAY

TO DO:

Task	Done
	☐
	☐
	☐
	☐
	☐
	☐
	☐
	☐
	☐
	☐

THURSDAY

FRIDAY

This Week's Affirmation:

It's all God who blesses me to do what I do.

Weekly Average Ticket Tracker

Knowing your average ticket tells you what each client is spending for their services and retail products.

Step1: Enter Your Info

Line 1: Total Service Dollar $_____
(enter the weekly amt. client spent only)

Line 2: Total Retail Dollars $_____
(enter the weekly amt. client spent only)

Line 3: Total # of Clients. _____
(enter the total amt. of clients serviced per week)

Step 2: Calculate The Information:

Line 4: Your Average Ticket. $_____
(take line 1 total service dollars and divide by the total # of clients from line 3).

Line 5: Your Average Retail Ticket $_____
(take line 2 your total retail dollars and divide by the total # of clients from line 3).

Base Price Budget Worksheet

Knowing your base price calculation will help you to structure your prices for your business and tells you what you need to charge each client in order to stay in business.

Follow the steps below to find out what is your Base Price Budget.

Step 1: Enter your information:

Line 1. Total Monthly Expense. $_____
*(enter all your **total monthly expenses**)*

Line 2. Projected Monthly Profit. $_____
*(enter the amount of profit **you want to make** Each month).*

Line 3. Total # Monthly Client Visits. _____
*(take the # of services you have, multiply by the # of clients **each person can serve in a month**. You can use your actual client count).*

Step 2: Now calculate the information below:

Line 4: Total projected gross sales $_____
*(take the **total monthly expenses** (line 1) and Add to the **projected monthly profit** (line 2).*

Line 5: Recommended base price
(take the total projected gross sales (line 4) $_____
*And divide the total # **monthly clients visits** (line 3).*

Notes

Slaying All Day!

MONDAY

TUESDAY

WEDNESDAY

THURSDAY

FRIDAY

WEEKEND

Goals
FOR THE WEEK

TO DO:

Task	Done
	☐
	☐
	☐
	☐
	☐
	☐
	☐
	☐
	☐
	☐

This Week's Affirmation:

I don't need permission to validate who I am.

Weekly Average Ticket Tracker

Knowing your average ticket tells you what each client is spending for their services and retail products.

Step1: Enter Your Info

Line 1: Total Service Dollar $_____
(enter the weekly amt. client spent only)

Line 2: Total Retail Dollars $_____
(enter the weekly amt. client spent only)

Line 3: Total # of Clients. _____
(enter the total amt. of clients serviced per week)

Step 2: Calculate The Information:

Line 4: Your Average Ticket. $_____
(take line 1 total service dollars and divide by the total # of clients from line 3).

Line 5: Your Average Retail Ticket $_____
(take line 2 your total retail dollars and divide by the total # of clients from line 3).

Base Price Budget Worksheet

Knowing your base price calculation will help you to structure your prices for your business and tells you what you need to charge each client in order to stay in business.

Follow the steps below to find out what is your Base Price Budget.

Step 1: Enter your information:

Line 1. Total Monthly Expense. $_____
*(enter all your **total monthly expenses**)*

Line 2. Projected Monthly Profit. $_____
*(enter the amount of profit **you want to make** Each month).*

Line 3. Total # Monthly Client Visits.   _____
*(take the # of services you have, multiply by the # of clients **each person can serve in a month**. You can use your actual client count).*

Step 2: Now calculate the information below:

Line 4: Total projected gross sales $_____
*(take the **total monthly expenses** (line 1) and Add to the **projected monthly profit** (line 2).*

Line 5: Recommended base price
(take the total projected gross sales (line 4) $_____
*And divide the total # **monthly clients visits** (line 3).*

Notes

Slaying All Day!

MONDAY

WEEKEND

TUESDAY

Goals
FOR THE WEEK

WEDNESDAY

TO DO:

Task	Done
	☐
	☐
	☐
	☐
	☐
	☐
	☐
	☐
	☐

THURSDAY

FRIDAY

This Week's Affirmation:

I will be bless others on my path.

Weekly Average Ticket Tracker

Knowing your average ticket tells you what each client is spending for their services and retail products.

Step1: Enter Your Info

Line 1: Total Service Dollar $_____
(enter the weekly amt. client spent only)

Line 2: Total Retail Dollars $_____
(enter the weekly amt. client spent only)

Line 3: Total # of Clients. _____
(enter the total amt. of clients serviced per week)

Step 2: Calculate The Information:

Line 4: Your Average Ticket. $_____
(take line 1 total service dollars and divide by the total # of clients from line 3).

Line 5: Your Average Retail Ticket $_____
(take line 2 your total retail dollars and divide by the total # of clients from line 3).

Base Price Budget Worksheet

Knowing your base price calculation will help you to structure your prices for your business and tells you what you need to charge each client in order to stay in business.

Follow the steps below to find out what is your Base Price Budget.

Step 1: Enter your information:

Line 1. Total Monthly Expense. $_____
*(enter all your **total monthly expenses**)*

Line 2. Projected Monthly Profit. $_____
*(enter the amount of profit **you want to make** Each month).*

Line 3. Total # Monthly Client Visits.   _____
*(take the # of services you have, multiply by the # of clients **each person can serve in a month**. You can use your actual client count).*

Step 2: Now calculate the information below:

Line 4: Total projected gross sales $_____
*(take the **total monthly expenses** (line 1) and Add to the **projected monthly profit** (line 2).*

Line 5: Recommended base price
*(take the total projected gross sales (line 4) $_____ And divide the total # **monthly clients visits** (line 3).*

Notes

Slaying All Day!

MONDAY

WEEKEND

TUESDAY

Goals
FOR THE WEEK

WEDNESDAY

THURSDAY

TO DO:

Task	Done
	☐
	☐
	☐
	☐
	☐
	☐
	☐
	☐
	☐

FRIDAY

This Week's Affirmation:

I claim health, prosperity and wealth in all areas of my life.

Weekly Average Ticket Tracker

Knowing your average ticket tells you what each client is spending for their services and retail products.

Step1: Enter Your Info

Line 1: Total Service Dollar $_____
(enter the weekly amt. client spent only)

Line 2: Total Retail Dollars $_____
(enter the weekly amt. client spent only)

Line 3: Total # of Clients. _____
(enter the total amt. of clients serviced per week)

Step 2: Calculate The Information:

Line 4: Your Average Ticket. $_____
(take line 1 total service dollars and divide by the total # of clients from line 3).

Line 5: Your Average Retail Ticket $_____
(take line 2 your total retail dollars and divide by the total # of clients from line 3).

Base Price Budget Worksheet

Knowing your base price calculation will help you to structure your prices for your business and tells you what you need to charge each client in order to stay in business.

Follow the steps below to find out what is your Base Price Budget.

Step 1: Enter your information:

Line 1. Total Monthly Expense. $_____
*(enter all your **total monthly expenses**)*

Line 2. Projected Monthly Profit. $_____
*(enter the amount of profit **you want to make** Each month).*

Line 3. Total # Monthly Client Visits.   _____
*(take the # of services you have, multiply by the # of clients **each person can serve in a month**. You can use your actual client count).*

Step 2: Now calculate the information below:

Line 4: Total projected gross sales $_____
*(take the **total monthly expenses** (line 1) and Add to the **projected monthly profit** (line 2).*

Line 5: Recommended base price
(take the total projected gross sales (line 4) $_____
*And divide the total # **monthly clients visits** (line 3).*

Notes

Slaying All Day!

MONDAY

WEEKEND

TUESDAY

Goals
FOR THE WEEK

WEDNESDAY

TO DO:

Task **Done**

THURSDAY

FRIDAY

This Week's Affirmation:

I am getting closer to my business goals each day.

Weekly Average Ticket Tracker

Knowing your average ticket tells you what each client is spending for their services and retail products.

Step1: Enter Your Info

**Line 1: Total Service Dollar $_____
(enter the weekly amt. client spent only)**

**Line 2: Total Retail Dollars $_____
(enter the weekly amt. client spent only)**

**Line 3: Total # of Clients. _____
(enter the total amt. of clients serviced per week)**

Step 2: Calculate The Information:

**Line 4: Your Average Ticket. $_____
(take line 1 total service dollars and divide by the total # of clients from line 3).**

**Line 5: Your Average Retail Ticket $_____
(take line 2 your total retail dollars and divide by the total # of clients from line 3).**

Base Price Budget Worksheet

Knowing your base price calculation will help you to structure your prices for your business and tells you what you need to charge each client in order to stay in business.

Follow the steps below to find out what is your Base Price Budget.

Step 1: Enter your information:

Line 1. Total Monthly Expense. $_____
*(enter all your **total monthly expenses**)*

Line 2. Projected Monthly Profit. $_____
*(enter the amount of profit **you want to make** Each month).*

Line 3. Total # Monthly Client Visits.   _____
*(take the # of services you have, multiply by the # of clients **each person can serve in a month**. You can use your actual client count).*

Step 2: Now calculate the information below:

Line 4: Total projected gross sales $_____
*(take the **total monthly expenses** (line 1) and Add to the **projected monthly profit** (line 2).*

Line 5: Recommended base price
(take the total projected gross sales (line 4) $_____
*And divide the total # **monthly clients visits** (line 3).*

Notes

Slaying All Day!

MONDAY

TUESDAY

WEDNESDAY

THURSDAY

FRIDAY

WEEKEND

Goals
FOR THE WEEK

TO DO:

Task	Done
	☐
	☐
	☐
	☐
	☐
	☐
	☐
	☐
	☐
	☐

This Week's Affirmation:

I will have multiple streams of income.

Weekly Average Ticket Tracker

Knowing your average ticket tells you what each client is spending for their services and retail products.

Step1: Enter Your Info

Line 1: Total Service Dollar $_____
(enter the weekly amt. client spent only)

Line 2: Total Retail Dollars $_____
(enter the weekly amt. client spent only)

Line 3: Total # of Clients. _____
(enter the total amt. of clients serviced per week)

Step 2: Calculate The Information:

Line 4: Your Average Ticket. $_____
(take line 1 total service dollars and divide by the total # of clients from line 3).

Line 5: Your Average Retail Ticket $_____
(take line 2 your total retail dollars and divide by the total # of clients from line 3).

Base Price Budget Worksheet

Knowing your base price calculation will help you to structure your prices for your business and tells you what you need to charge each client in order to stay in business.

Follow the steps below to find out what is your Base Price Budget.

Step 1: Enter your information:

Line 1. Total Monthly Expense. $_____
*(enter all your **total monthly expenses**)*

Line 2. Projected Monthly Profit. $_____
*(enter the amount of profit **you want to make** Each month).*

Line 3. Total # Monthly Client Visits.   _____
*(take the # of services you have, multiply by the # of clients **each person can serve in a month**. You can use your actual client count).*

Step 2: Now calculate the information below:

Line 4: Total projected gross sales $_____
*(take the **total monthly expenses** (line 1) and Add to the **projected monthly profit** (line 2).*

Line 5: Recommended base price
(take the total projected gross sales (line 4) $_____
*And divide the total # **monthly clients visits** (line 3).*

Notes

Slaying All Day!

MONDAY

WEEKEND

TUESDAY

Goals
FOR THE WEEK

WEDNESDAY

TO DO:

Task   **Done**

THURSDAY

FRIDAY

This Week's Affirmation:

I am a winner and I will never give up on pursuing my dreams.

Weekly Average Ticket Tracker

Knowing your average ticket tells you what each client is spending for their services and retail products.

Step1: Enter Your Info

Line 1: Total Service Dollar $_______________
(enter the weekly amt. client spent only)

Line 2: Total Retail Dollars $_______________
(enter the weekly amt. client spent only)

Line 3: Total # of Clients. __________________
(enter the total amt. of clients serviced per week)

Step 2: Calculate The Information:

Line 4: Your Average Ticket. $_______________
(take line 1 total service dollars and divide by the total # of clients from line 3).

Line 5: Your Average Retail Ticket $_____________
(take line 2 your total retail dollars and divide by the total # of clients from line 3).

Base Price Budget Worksheet

Knowing your base price calculation will help you to structure your prices for your business and tells you what you need to charge each client in order to stay in business.

Follow the steps below to find out what is your Base Price Budget.

Step 1: Enter your information:

Line 1. Total Monthly Expense. $_____
*(enter all your **total monthly expenses**)*

Line 2. Projected Monthly Profit. $_____
*(enter the amount of profit **you want to make** Each month).*

Line 3. Total # Monthly Client Visits.   _____
*(take the # of services you have, multiply by the # of clients **each person can serve in a month**. You can use your actual client count).*

Step 2: Now calculate the information below:

Line 4: Total projected gross sales $_____
*(take the **total monthly expenses** (line 1) and Add to the **projected monthly profit** (line 2).*

Line 5: Recommended base price
(take the total projected gross sales (line 4) $_____
*And divide the total # **monthly clients visits** (line 3).*

Notes

Slaying All Day!

MONDAY

WEEKEND

TUESDAY

Goals FOR THE WEEK

WEDNESDAY

THURSDAY

TO DO:

Task	Done
	☐
	☐
	☐
	☐
	☐
	☐
	☐
	☐

FRIDAY

This Week's Affirmation:

I am grateful for every business opportunity

Weekly Average Ticket Tracker

Knowing your average ticket tells you what each client is spending for their services and retail products.

Step1: Enter Your Info

Line 1: Total Service Dollar $_____
(enter the weekly amt. client spent only)

Line 2: Total Retail Dollars $_____
(enter the weekly amt. client spent only)

Line 3: Total # of Clients. _____
(enter the total amt. of clients serviced per week)

Step 2: Calculate The Information:

Line 4: Your Average Ticket. $_____
(take line 1 total service dollars and divide by the total # of clients from line 3).

Line 5: Your Average Retail Ticket $_____
(take line 2 your total retail dollars and divide by the total # of clients from line 3).

Base Price Budget Worksheet

Knowing your base price calculation will help you to structure your prices for your business and tells you what you need to charge each client in order to stay in business.

Follow the steps below to find out what is your Base Price Budget.

Step 1: Enter your information:

Line 1. Total Monthly Expense. $_____
*(enter all your **total monthly expenses**)*

Line 2. Projected Monthly Profit. $_____
*(enter the amount of profit **you want to make**
Each month).*

Line 3. Total # Monthly Client Visits.   _____
*(take the # of services you have, multiply by the
# of clients **each person can serve in a month**.
You can use your actual client count).*

Step 2: Now calculate the information below:

Line 4: Total projected gross sales $_____
*(take the **total monthly expenses** (line 1) and
Add to the **projected monthly profit** (line 2).*

Line 5: Recommended base price
(take the total projected gross sales (line 4) $_____
*And divide the total # **monthly clients visits**
(line 3).*

Notes

Slaying All Day!

DATE

__ / __ / __

MONDAY

WEEKEND

TUESDAY

Goals
FOR THE WEEK

WEDNESDAY

TO DO:

Task	Done
	☐
	☐
	☐
	☐
	☐
	☐
	☐
	☐
	☐

THURSDAY

FRIDAY

This Week's Affirmation:

My heart is open to receive the blessings of God.

Weekly Average Ticket Tracker

Knowing your average ticket tells you what each client is spending for their services and retail products.

Step1: Enter Your Info

Line 1: Total Service Dollar $_____
(enter the weekly amt. client spent only)

Line 2: Total Retail Dollars $_____
(enter the weekly amt. client spent only)

Line 3: Total # of Clients. _____
(enter the total amt. of clients serviced per week)

Step 2: Calculate The Information:

Line 4: Your Average Ticket. $_____
(take line 1 total service dollars and divide by the total # of clients from line 3).

Line 5: Your Average Retail Ticket $_____
(take line 2 your total retail dollars and divide by the total # of clients from line 3).

Base Price Budget Worksheet

Knowing your base price calculation will help you to structure your prices for your business and tells you what you need to charge each client in order to stay in business.

Follow the steps below to find out what is your Base Price Budget.

Step 1: Enter your information:

Line 1. Total Monthly Expense. $_____
*(enter all your **total monthly expenses**)*

Line 2. Projected Monthly Profit. $_____
*(enter the amount of profit **you want to make** Each month).*

Line 3. Total # Monthly Client Visits.   _____
*(take the # of services you have, multiply by the # of clients **each person can serve in a month**. You can use your actual client count).*

Step 2: Now calculate the information below:

Line 4: Total projected gross sales $_____
*(take the **total monthly expenses** (line 1) and Add to the **projected monthly profit** (line 2).*

Line 5: Recommended base price
*(take the total projected gross sales (line 4) $_____ And divide the total # **monthly clients visits** (line 3).*

Notes

Slaying All Day!

DATE
__ / __ / __

MONDAY

WEEKEND

TUESDAY

Goals
FOR THE WEEK

WEDNESDAY

TO DO:

Task   **Done**

☐
☐
☐
☐
☐
☐
☐
☐
☐
☐

THURSDAY

FRIDAY

This Week's Affirmation:

I invest in the best and expect the same in return.

Weekly Average Ticket Tracker

Knowing your average ticket tells you what each client is spending for their services and retail products.

Step1: Enter Your Info

Line 1: Total Service Dollar $_____
(enter the weekly amt. client spent only)

Line 2: Total Retail Dollars $_____
(enter the weekly amt. client spent only)

Line 3: Total # of Clients. _____
(enter the total amt. of clients serviced per week)

Step 2: Calculate The Information:

Line 4: Your Average Ticket. $_____
(take line 1 total service dollars and divide by the total # of clients from line 3).

Line 5: Your Average Retail Ticket $_____
(take line 2 your total retail dollars and divide by the total # of clients from line 3).

Base Price Budget Worksheet

Knowing your base price calculation will help you to structure your prices for your business and tells you what you need to charge each client in order to stay in business.

Follow the steps below to find out what is your Base Price Budget.

Step 1: Enter your information:

Line 1. Total Monthly Expense. $_____
*(enter all your **total monthly expenses**)*

Line 2. Projected Monthly Profit. $_____
*(enter the amount of profit **you want to make** Each month).*

Line 3. Total # Monthly Client Visits.   _____
*(take the # of services you have, multiply by the # of clients **each person can serve in a month**. You can use your actual client count).*

Step 2: Now calculate the information below:

Line 4: Total projected gross sales $_____
*(take the **total monthly expenses** (line 1) and Add to the **projected monthly profit** (line 2).*

Line 5: Recommended base price
*(take the total projected gross sales (line 4) $_____
And divide the total # **monthly clients visits** (line 3).*

Notes

Slaying All Day!

MONDAY

WEEKEND

TUESDAY

Goals FOR THE WEEK

WEDNESDAY

THURSDAY

TO DO:

Task	Done
	☐
	☐
	☐
	☐
	☐
	☐
	☐
	☐
	☐
	☐

FRIDAY

This Week's Affirmation:

I am unstoppable.

Weekly Average Ticket Tracker

Knowing your average ticket tells you what each client is spending for their services and retail products.

Step1: Enter Your Info

Line 1: Total Service Dollar $_____
(enter the weekly amt. client spent only)

Line 2: Total Retail Dollars $_____
(enter the weekly amt. client spent only)

Line 3: Total # of Clients. _____
(enter the total amt. of clients serviced per week)

Step 2: Calculate The Information:

Line 4: Your Average Ticket. $_____
(take line 1 total service dollars and divide by the total # of clients from line 3).

Line 5: Your Average Retail Ticket $_____
(take line 2 your total retail dollars and divide by the total # of clients from line 3).

Base Price Budget Worksheet

Knowing your base price calculation will help you to structure your prices for your business and tells you what you need to charge each client in order to stay in business.

Follow the steps below to find out what is your Base Price Budget.

Step 1: Enter your information:

Line 1. Total Monthly Expense. $_____
*(enter all your **total monthly expenses**)*

Line 2. Projected Monthly Profit. $_____
*(enter the amount of profit **you want to make** Each month).*

Line 3. Total # Monthly Client Visits.   _____
*(take the # of services you have, multiply by the # of clients **each person can serve in a month**. You can use your actual client count).*

Step 2: Now calculate the information below:

Line 4: Total projected gross sales $_____
*(take the **total monthly expenses** (line 1) and Add to the **projected monthly profit** (line 2).*

Line 5: Recommended base price
(take the total projected gross sales (line 4) $_____
*And divide the total # **monthly clients visits** (line 3).*

Notes

Slaying All Day!

MONDAY

WEEKEND

TUESDAY

Goals
FOR THE WEEK

WEDNESDAY

TO DO:

Task	Done
	☐
	☐
	☐
	☐
	☐
	☐
	☐
	☐
	☐
	☐

THURSDAY

FRIDAY

This Week's Affirmation:

I am capable of amazing things.

Weekly Average Ticket Tracker

Knowing your average ticket tells you what each client is spending for their services and retail products.

Step1: Enter Your Info

**Line 1: Total Service Dollar $_____
(enter the weekly amt. client spent only)**

**Line 2: Total Retail Dollars $_____
(enter the weekly amt. client spent only)**

**Line 3: Total # of Clients. _____
(enter the total amt. of clients serviced per week)**

Step 2: Calculate The Information:

**Line 4: Your Average Ticket. $_____
(take line 1 total service dollars and divide by the total # of clients from line 3).**

**Line 5: Your Average Retail Ticket $_____
(take line 2 your total retail dollars and divide by the total # of clients from line 3).**

Base Price Budget Worksheet

Knowing your base price calculation will help you to structure your prices for your business and tells you what you need to charge each client in order to stay in business.

Follow the steps below to find out what is your Base Price Budget.

Step 1: Enter your information:

Line 1. Total Monthly Expense. $_____
*(enter all your **total monthly expenses**)*

Line 2. Projected Monthly Profit. $_____
*(enter the amount of profit **you want to make** Each month).*

Line 3. Total # Monthly Client Visits. _____
*(take the # of services you have, multiply by the # of clients **each person can serve in a month**. You can use your actual client count).*

Step 2: Now calculate the information below:

Line 4: Total projected gross sales $_____
*(take the **total monthly expenses** (line 1) and Add to the **projected monthly profit** (line 2).*

Line 5: Recommended base price
(take the total projected gross sales (line 4) $_____
*And divide the total # **monthly clients visits** (line 3).*

Notes

Slaying All Day!

MONDAY

WEEKEND

TUESDAY

Goals
FOR THE WEEK

WEDNESDAY

TO DO:

Task	Done
	☐
	☐
	☐
	☐
	☐
	☐
	☐
	☐
	☐
	☐

THURSDAY

FRIDAY

This Week's Affirmation:

I am more than enough.

Weekly Average Ticket Tracker

Knowing your average ticket tells you what each client is spending for their services and retail products.

Step1: Enter Your Info

Line 1: Total Service Dollar $_____
(enter the weekly amt. client spent only)

Line 2: Total Retail Dollars $_____
(enter the weekly amt. client spent only)

Line 3: Total # of Clients. _____
(enter the total amt. of clients serviced per week)

Step 2: Calculate The Information:

Line 4: Your Average Ticket. $_____
(take line 1 total service dollars and divide by the total # of clients from line 3).

Line 5: Your Average Retail Ticket $_____
(take line 2 your total retail dollars and divide by the total # of clients from line 3).

Base Price Budget Worksheet

Knowing your base price calculation will help you to structure your prices for your business and tells you what you need to charge each client in order to stay in business.

Follow the steps below to find out what is your Base Price Budget.

Step 1: Enter your information:

Line 1. Total Monthly Expense. $_____
*(enter all your **total monthly expenses**)*

Line 2. Projected Monthly Profit. $_____
*(enter the amount of profit **you want to make** Each month).*

Line 3. Total # Monthly Client Visits. _____
*(take the # of services you have, multiply by the # of clients **each person can serve in a month**. You can use your actual client count).*

Step 2: Now calculate the information below:

Line 4: Total projected gross sales $_____
*(take the **total monthly expenses** (line 1) and Add to the **projected monthly profit** (line 2).*

Line 5: Recommended base price
(take the total projected gross sales (line 4) $_____
*And divide the total # **monthly clients visits** (line 3).*

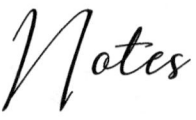

Notes

Slaying All Day!

MONDAY

TUESDAY

WEDNESDAY

THURSDAY

FRIDAY

WEEKEND

Goals
FOR THE WEEK

TO DO:

Task	Done
	☐
	☐
	☐
	☐
	☐
	☐
	☐
	☐
	☐

This Week's Affirmation:

This is my year of love, peace, joy and abundant living.

Weekly Average Ticket Tracker

Knowing your average ticket tells you what each client is spending for their services and retail products.

Step1: Enter Your Info

Line 1: Total Service Dollar $_____
(enter the weekly amt. client spent only)

Line 2: Total Retail Dollars $_____
(enter the weekly amt. client spent only)

Line 3: Total # of Clients. _____
(enter the total amt. of clients serviced per week)

Step 2: Calculate The Information:

Line 4: Your Average Ticket. $_____
(take line 1 total service dollars and divide by the total # of clients from line 3).

Line 5: Your Average Retail Ticket $_____
(take line 2 your total retail dollars and divide by the total # of clients from line 3).

Base Price Budget Worksheet

Knowing your base price calculation will help you to structure your prices for your business and tells you what you need to charge each client in order to stay in business.

Follow the steps below to find out what is your Base Price Budget.

Step 1: Enter your information:

Line 1. Total Monthly Expense. $_____
(enter all your **total monthly expenses**)

Line 2. Projected Monthly Profit. $_____
(enter the amount of profit **you want to make** Each month).

Line 3. Total # Monthly Client Visits.   _____
(take the # of services you have, multiply by the # of clients **each person can serve in a month**. You can use your actual client count).

Step 2: Now calculate the information below:

Line 4: Total projected gross sales $_____
(take the **total monthly expenses** (line 1) and Add to the **projected monthly profit** (line 2).

Line 5: Recommended base price
(take the total projected gross sales (line 4) $_____
And divide the total # **monthly clients visits** (line 3).

Notes

Slaying All Day!

MONDAY

WEEKEND

TUESDAY

Goals
FOR THE WEEK

WEDNESDAY

THURSDAY

TO DO:

Task	Done
	☐
	☐
	☐
	☐
	☐
	☐
	☐
	☐
	☐
	☐

FRIDAY

This Week's Affirmation:

I am working on the change I want to see.

Weekly Average Ticket Tracker

Knowing your average ticket tells you what each client is spending for their services and retail products.

Step1: Enter Your Info

Line 1: Total Service Dollar $_____
(enter the weekly amt. client spent only)

Line 2: Total Retail Dollars $_____
(enter the weekly amt. client spent only)

Line 3: Total # of Clients. _____
(enter the total amt. of clients serviced per week)

Step 2: Calculate The Information:

Line 4: Your Average Ticket. $_____
(take line 1 total service dollars and divide by the total # of clients from line 3).

Line 5: Your Average Retail Ticket $_____
(take line 2 your total retail dollars and divide by the total # of clients from line 3).

Base Price Budget Worksheet

Knowing your base price calculation will help you to structure your prices for your business and tells you what you need to charge each client in order to stay in business.

Follow the steps below to find out what is your Base Price Budget.

Step 1: Enter your information:

Line 1. Total Monthly Expense. $_____
*(enter all your **total monthly expenses**)*

Line 2. Projected Monthly Profit. $_____
*(enter the amount of profit **you want to make** Each month).*

Line 3. Total # Monthly Client Visits.   _____
*(take the # of services you have, multiply by the # of clients **each person can serve in a month**. You can use your actual client count).*

Step 2: Now calculate the information below:

Line 4: Total projected gross sales $_____
*(take the **total monthly expenses** (line 1) and Add to the **projected monthly profit** (line 2).*

Line 5: Recommended base price
*(take the total projected gross sales (line 4) $_____
And divide the total # **monthly clients visits** (line 3).*

Notes

Slaying All Day!

MONDAY

WEEKEND

TUESDAY

Goals
FOR THE WEEK

WEDNESDAY

TO DO:

Task	Done
	☐
	☐
	☐
	☐
	☐
	☐
	☐
	☐
	☐
	☐

THURSDAY

FRIDAY

This Week's Affirmation:

My day is filled with unlimited possibilities.

Weekly Average Ticket Tracker

Knowing your average ticket tells you what each client is spending for their services and retail products.

Step1: Enter Your Info

Line 1: Total Service Dollar $_____
(enter the weekly amt. client spent only)

Line 2: Total Retail Dollars $_____
(enter the weekly amt. client spent only)

Line 3: Total # of Clients. _____
(enter the total amt. of clients serviced per week)

Step 2: Calculate The Information:

Line 4: Your Average Ticket. $_____
(take line 1 total service dollars and divide by the total # of clients from line 3).

Line 5: Your Average Retail Ticket $_____
(take line 2 your total retail dollars and divide by the total # of clients from line 3).

Base Price Budget Worksheet

Knowing your base price calculation will help you to structure your prices for your business and tells you what you need to charge each client in order to stay in business.

Follow the steps below to find out what is your Base Price Budget.

Step 1: Enter your information:

Line 1. Total Monthly Expense. $_____
*(enter all your **total monthly expenses**)*

Line 2. Projected Monthly Profit. $_____
*(enter the amount of profit **you want to make**
Each month).*

Line 3. Total # Monthly Client Visits.   _____
*(take the # of services you have, multiply by the
# of clients **each person can serve in a month**.
You can use your actual client count).*

Step 2: Now calculate the information below:

Line 4: Total projected gross sales $_____
*(take the **total monthly expenses** (line 1) and
Add to the **projected monthly profit** (line 2).*

Line 5: Recommended base price
(take the total projected gross sales (line 4) $_____
*And divide the total # **monthly clients visits**
(line 3).*

Notes

Slaying All Day!

MONDAY

WEEKEND

TUESDAY

Goals
FOR THE WEEK

WEDNESDAY

TO DO:

Task	Done
	☐
	☐
	☐
	☐
	☐
	☐
	☐
	☐
	☐

THURSDAY

FRIDAY

This Week's Affirmation:

I have the power from within to be successful.

Weekly Average Ticket Tracker

Knowing your average ticket tells you what each client is spending for their services and retail products.

Step1: Enter Your Info

Line 1: Total Service Dollar $_____
(enter the weekly amt. client spent only)

Line 2: Total Retail Dollars $_____
(enter the weekly amt. client spent only)

Line 3: Total # of Clients. _____
(enter the total amt. of clients serviced per week)

Step 2: Calculate The Information:

Line 4: Your Average Ticket. $_____
(take line 1 total service dollars and divide by the total # of clients from line 3).

Line 5: Your Average Retail Ticket $_____
(take line 2 your total retail dollars and divide by the total # of clients from line 3).

Base Price Budget Worksheet

Knowing your base price calculation will help you to structure your prices for your business and tells you what you need to charge each client in order to stay in business.

Follow the steps below to find out what is your Base Price Budget.

Step 1: Enter your information:

Line 1. Total Monthly Expense. $_____
*(enter all your **total monthly expenses**)*

Line 2. Projected Monthly Profit. $_____
*(enter the amount of profit **you want to make** Each month).*

Line 3. Total # Monthly Client Visits.   _____
*(take the # of services you have, multiply by the # of clients **each person can serve in a month**. You can use your actual client count).*

Step 2: Now calculate the information below:

Line 4: Total projected gross sales $_____
*(take the **total monthly expenses** (line 1) and Add to the **projected monthly profit** (line 2).*

Line 5: Recommended base price
(take the total projected gross sales (line 4) $_____
*And divide the total # **monthly clients visits** (line 3).*

Notes

Slaying All Day!

MONDAY

WEEKEND

TUESDAY

Goals
FOR THE WEEK

WEDNESDAY

TO DO:

Task	Done
	☐
	☐
	☐
	☐
	☐
	☐
	☐
	☐
	☐
	☐

THURSDAY

FRIDAY

This Week's Affirmation:

Today I will show an attitude of gratitude.

Weekly Average Ticket Tracker

Knowing your average ticket tells you what each client is spending for their services and retail products.

Step1: Enter Your Info

Line 1: Total Service Dollar $_____
(enter the weekly amt. client spent only)

Line 2: Total Retail Dollars $_____
(enter the weekly amt. client spent only)

Line 3: Total # of Clients. _____
(enter the total amt. of clients serviced per week)

Step 2: Calculate The Information:

Line 4: Your Average Ticket. $_____
(take line 1 total service dollars and divide by the total # of clients from line 3).

Line 5: Your Average Retail Ticket $_____
(take line 2 your total retail dollars and divide by the total # of clients from line 3).

Base Price Budget Worksheet

Knowing your base price calculation will help you to structure your prices for your business and tells you what you need to charge each client in order to stay in business.

Follow the steps below to find out what is your Base Price Budget.

Step 1: Enter your information:

Line 1. Total Monthly Expense. $_____
*(enter all your **total monthly expenses**)*

Line 2. Projected Monthly Profit. $_____
*(enter the amount of profit **you want to make** Each month).*

Line 3. Total # Monthly Client Visits.   _____
*(take the # of services you have, multiply by the # of clients **each person can serve in a month**. You can use your actual client count).*

Step 2: Now calculate the information below:

Line 4: Total projected gross sales $_____
*(take the **total monthly expenses** (line 1) and Add to the **projected monthly profit** (line 2).*

Line 5: Recommended base price
(take the total projected gross sales (line 4) $_____
*And divide the total # **monthly clients visits** (line 3).*

Notes

Slaying All Day!

DATE

__ __ / __ __ / __ __

MONDAY

WEEKEND

TUESDAY

Goals
FOR THE WEEK

WEDNESDAY

TO DO:

Task	Done
	☐
	☐
	☐
	☐
	☐
	☐
	☐
	☐
	☐
	☐

THURSDAY

FRIDAY

This Week's Affirmation:

I am thankful for my past that set me up for my present.

Weekly Average Ticket Tracker

Knowing your average ticket tells you what each client is spending for their services and retail products.

Step1: Enter Your Info

Line 1: Total Service Dollar $_____
(enter the weekly amt. client spent only)

Line 2: Total Retail Dollars $_____
(enter the weekly amt. client spent only)

Line 3: Total # of Clients. _____
(enter the total amt. of clients serviced per week)

Step 2: Calculate The Information:

Line 4: Your Average Ticket. $_____
(take line 1 total service dollars and divide by the total # of clients from line 3).

Line 5: Your Average Retail Ticket $_____
(take line 2 your total retail dollars and divide by the total # of clients from line 3).

Knowing your base price calculation will help you to structure your prices for your business and tells you what you need to charge each client in order to stay in business.

Follow the steps below to find out what is your Base Price Budget.

Step 1: Enter your information:

Line 1. Total Monthly Expense. $_____
*(enter all your **total monthly expenses**)*

Line 2. Projected Monthly Profit. $_____
*(enter the amount of profit **you want to make** Each month).*

Line 3. Total # Monthly Client Visits.   _____
*(take the # of services you have, multiply by the # of clients **each person can serve in a month**. You can use your actual client count).*

Step 2: Now calculate the information below:

Line 4: Total projected gross sales $_____
*(take the **total monthly expenses** (line 1) and Add to the **projected monthly profit** (line 2).*

Line 5: Recommended base price
(take the total projected gross sales (line 4) $_____
*And divide the total # **monthly clients visits** (line 3).*

Notes

Slaying All Day!

DATE

__ / __ / __

MONDAY

WEEKEND

TUESDAY

Goals
FOR THE WEEK

WEDNESDAY

THURSDAY

TO DO:

Task	Done
	☐
	☐
	☐
	☐
	☐
	☐
	☐
	☐
	☐
	☐

FRIDAY

This Week's Affirmation:

I will not stress over things not in my control.

Weekly Average Ticket Tracker

Knowing your average ticket tells you what each client is spending for their services and retail products.

Step1: Enter Your Info

Line 1: Total Service Dollar $_____
(enter the weekly amt. client spent only)

Line 2: Total Retail Dollars $_____
(enter the weekly amt. client spent only)

Line 3: Total # of Clients. _____
(enter the total amt. of clients serviced per week)

Step 2: Calculate The Information:

Line 4: Your Average Ticket. $_____
(take line 1 total service dollars and divide by the total # of clients from line 3).

Line 5: Your Average Retail Ticket $_____
(take line 2 your total retail dollars and divide by the total # of clients from line 3).

Base Price Budget Worksheet

Knowing your base price calculation will help you to structure your prices for your business and tells you what you need to charge each client in order to stay in business.

Follow the steps below to find out what is your Base Price Budget.

Step 1: Enter your information:

Line 1. Total Monthly Expense. $_____
*(enter all your **total monthly expenses**)*

Line 2. Projected Monthly Profit. $_____
*(enter the amount of profit **you want to make** Each month).*

Line 3. Total # Monthly Client Visits.   _____
*(take the # of services you have, multiply by the # of clients **each person can serve in a month**. You can use your actual client count).*

Step 2: Now calculate the information below:

Line 4: Total projected gross sales $_____
*(take the **total monthly expenses** (line 1) and Add to the **projected monthly profit** (line 2).*

Line 5: Recommended base price
(take the total projected gross sales (line 4) $_____
*And divide the total # **monthly clients visits** (line 3).*

Notes

Slaying All Day!

MONDAY

WEEKEND

TUESDAY

Goals
FOR THE WEEK

WEDNESDAY

THURSDAY

TO DO:

Task   **Done**

FRIDAY

This Week's Affirmation:

Be still and know there's a solution to every challenge.

Weekly Average Ticket Tracker

Knowing your average ticket tells you what each client is spending for their services and retail products.

Step1: Enter Your Info

Line 1: Total Service Dollar $_____
(enter the weekly amt. client spent only)

Line 2: Total Retail Dollars $_____
(enter the weekly amt. client spent only)

Line 3: Total # of Clients. _____
(enter the total amt. of clients serviced per week)

Step 2: Calculate The Information:

Line 4: Your Average Ticket. $_____
(take line 1 total service dollars and divide by the total # of clients from line 3).

Line 5: Your Average Retail Ticket $_____
(take line 2 your total retail dollars and divide by the total # of clients from line 3).

Base Price Budget Worksheet

Knowing your base price calculation will help you to structure your prices for your business and tells you what you need to charge each client in order to stay in business.

Follow the steps below to find out what is your Base Price Budget.

Step 1: Enter your information:

Line 1. Total Monthly Expense. $_____
*(enter all your **total monthly expenses**)*

Line 2. Projected Monthly Profit. $_____
*(enter the amount of profit **you want to make** Each month).*

Line 3. Total # Monthly Client Visits.   _____
*(take the # of services you have, multiply by the # of clients **each person can serve in a month**. You can use your actual client count).*

Step 2: Now calculate the information below:

Line 4: Total projected gross sales $_____
*(take the **total monthly expenses** (line 1) and Add to the **projected monthly profit** (line 2).*

Line 5: Recommended base price
(take the total projected gross sales (line 4) $_____
*And divide the total # **monthly clients visits** (line 3).*

Notes

Slaying All Day!

DATE

__ __ / __ __ / __ __

MONDAY

WEEKEND

TUESDAY

Goals
FOR THE WEEK

WEDNESDAY

TO DO:

Task	Done
	☐
	☐
	☐
	☐
	☐
	☐
	☐
	☐
	☐
	☐

THURSDAY

FRIDAY

This Week's Affirmation:

Seek ways to elevate your customer service.

Weekly Average Ticket Tracker

Knowing your average ticket tells you what each client is spending for their services and retail products.

Step1: Enter Your Info

Line 1: Total Service Dollar $_____
(enter the weekly amt. client spent only)

Line 2: Total Retail Dollars $_____
(enter the weekly amt. client spent only)

Line 3: Total # of Clients. _____
(enter the total amt. of clients serviced per week)

Step 2: Calculate The Information:

Line 4: Your Average Ticket. $_____
(take line 1 total service dollars and divide by the total # of clients from line 3).

Line 5: Your Average Retail Ticket $_____
(take line 2 your total retail dollars and divide by the total # of clients from line 3).

Base Price Budget Worksheet

Knowing your base price calculation will help you to structure your prices for your business and tells you what you need to charge each client in order to stay in business.

Follow the steps below to find out what is your Base Price Budget.

Step 1: Enter your information:

Line 1. Total Monthly Expense. $_____
*(enter all your **total monthly expenses**)*

Line 2. Projected Monthly Profit. $_____
*(enter the amount of profit **you want to make**
Each month).*

Line 3. Total # Monthly Client Visits.   _____
*(take the # of services you have, multiply by the
# of clients **each person can serve in a month**.
You can use your actual client count).*

Step 2: Now calculate the information below:

Line 4: Total projected gross sales $_____
*(take the **total monthly expenses** (line 1) and
Add to the **projected monthly profit** (line 2).*

Line 5: Recommended base price
(take the total projected gross sales (line 4) $_____
*And divide the total # **monthly clients visits**
(line 3).*

Notes

Slaying All Day!

MONDAY

WEEKEND

TUESDAY

Goals
FOR THE WEEK

WEDNESDAY

TO DO:

Task	Done
	☐
	☐
	☐
	☐
	☐
	☐
	☐
	☐
	☐
	☐

THURSDAY

FRIDAY

This Week's Affirmation:

Set yourself apart from being average.

Weekly Average Ticket Tracker

Knowing your average ticket tells you what each client is spending for their services and retail products.

Step1: Enter Your Info

Line 1: Total Service Dollar $_____
(enter the weekly amt. client spent only)

Line 2: Total Retail Dollars $_____
(enter the weekly amt. client spent only)

Line 3: Total # of Clients. _____
(enter the total amt. of clients serviced per week)

Step 2: Calculate The Information:

Line 4: Your Average Ticket. $_____
(take line 1 total service dollars and divide by the total # of clients from line 3).

Line 5: Your Average Retail Ticket $_____
(take line 2 your total retail dollars and divide by the total # of clients from line 3).

Base Price Budget Worksheet

Knowing your base price calculation will help you to structure your prices for your business and tells you what you need to charge each client in order to stay in business.

Follow the steps below to find out what is your Base Price Budget.

Step 1: Enter your information:

Line 1. Total Monthly Expense. $_____
*(enter all your **total monthly expenses**)*

Line 2. Projected Monthly Profit. $_____
*(enter the amount of profit **you want to make** Each month).*

Line 3. Total # Monthly Client Visits. _____
*(take the # of services you have, multiply by the # of clients **each person can serve in a month**. You can use your actual client count).*

Step 2: Now calculate the information below:

Line 4: Total projected gross sales $_____
*(take the **total monthly expenses** (line 1) and Add to the **projected monthly profit** (line 2).*

Line 5: Recommended base price
(take the total projected gross sales (line 4) $_____
*And divide the total # **monthly clients visits** (line 3).*

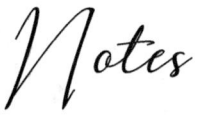

Notes

Slaying All Day!

MONDAY

WEEKEND

TUESDAY

Goals
FOR THE WEEK

WEDNESDAY

TO DO:

Task	Done
	☐
	☐
	☐
	☐
	☐
	☐
	☐
	☐
	☐
	☐

THURSDAY

FRIDAY

This Week's Affirmation:

Always keep a positive attitude even in crappy situations.

Weekly Average Ticket Tracker

Knowing your average ticket tells you what each client is spending for their services and retail products.

Step1: Enter Your Info

Line 1: Total Service Dollar $_____
(enter the weekly amt. client spent only)

Line 2: Total Retail Dollars $_____
(enter the weekly amt. client spent only)

Line 3: Total # of Clients. _____
(enter the total amt. of clients serviced per week)

Step 2: Calculate The Information:

Line 4: Your Average Ticket. $_____
(take line 1 total service dollars and divide by the total # of clients from line 3).

Line 5: Your Average Retail Ticket $_____
(take line 2 your total retail dollars and divide by the total # of clients from line 3).

Base Price Budget Worksheet

Knowing your base price calculation will help you to structure your prices for your business and tells you what you need to charge each client in order to stay in business.

Follow the steps below to find out what is your Base Price Budget.

Step 1: Enter your information:

Line 1. Total Monthly Expense. $_____
*(enter all your **total monthly expenses**)*

Line 2. Projected Monthly Profit. $_____
*(enter the amount of profit **you want to make** Each month).*

Line 3. Total # Monthly Client Visits.   _____
*(take the # of services you have, multiply by the # of clients **each person can serve in a month**. You can use your actual client count).*

Step 2: Now calculate the information below:

Line 4: Total projected gross sales $_____
*(take the **total monthly expenses** (line 1) and Add to the **projected monthly profit** (line 2).*

Line 5: Recommended base price
(take the total projected gross sales (line 4) $_____
*And divide the total # **monthly clients visits** (line 3).*

Notes

Slaying All Day!

MONDAY

WEEKEND

TUESDAY

Goals
FOR THE WEEK

WEDNESDAY

TO DO:

Task	Done
	☐
	☐
	☐
	☐
	☐
	☐
	☐
	☐
	☐
	☐

THURSDAY

FRIDAY

This Week's Affirmation:

Be a Boss that elevates others.

Weekly Average Ticket Tracker

Knowing your average ticket tells you what each client is spending for their services and retail products.

Step1: Enter Your Info

Line 1: Total Service Dollar $_____
(enter the weekly amt. client spent only)

Line 2: Total Retail Dollars $_____
(enter the weekly amt. client spent only)

Line 3: Total # of Clients. _____
(enter the total amt. of clients serviced per week)

Step 2: Calculate The Information:

Line 4: Your Average Ticket. $_____
(take line 1 total service dollars and divide by the total # of clients from line 3).

Line 5: Your Average Retail Ticket $_____
(take line 2 your total retail dollars and divide by the total # of clients from line 3).

Base Price Budget Worksheet

Knowing your base price calculation will help you to structure your prices for your business and tells you what you need to charge each client in order to stay in business.

Follow the steps below to find out what is your Base Price Budget.

Step 1: Enter your information:

Line 1. Total Monthly Expense. $_____
*(enter all your **total monthly expenses**)*

Line 2. Projected Monthly Profit. $_____
*(enter the amount of profit **you want to make** Each month).*

Line 3. Total # Monthly Client Visits.   _____
*(take the # of services you have, multiply by the # of clients **each person can serve in a month**. You can use your actual client count).*

Step 2: Now calculate the information below:

Line 4: Total projected gross sales $_____
*(take the **total monthly expenses** (line 1) and Add to the **projected monthly profit** (line 2).*

Line 5: Recommended base price
(take the total projected gross sales (line 4) $_____
*And divide the total # **monthly clients visits** (line 3).*

Notes

Slaying All Day!

MONDAY

WEEKEND

TUESDAY

Goals
FOR THE WEEK

WEDNESDAY

TO DO:

Task	Done
	☐
	☐
	☐
	☐
	☐
	☐
	☐
	☐
	☐
	☐

THURSDAY

FRIDAY

This Week's Affirmation:

Aim to deliver an extraordinary experience.

Weekly Average Ticket Tracker

Knowing your average ticket tells you what each client is spending for their services and retail products.

Step1: Enter Your Info

Line 1: Total Service Dollar $_____
(enter the weekly amt. client spent only)

Line 2: Total Retail Dollars $_____
(enter the weekly amt. client spent only)

Line 3: Total # of Clients. _____
(enter the total amt. of clients serviced per week)

Step 2: Calculate The Information:

Line 4: Your Average Ticket. $_____
(take line 1 total service dollars and divide by the total # of clients from line 3).

Line 5: Your Average Retail Ticket $_____
(take line 2 your total retail dollars and divide by the total # of clients from line 3).

Base Price Budget Worksheet

Knowing your base price calculation will help you to structure your prices for your business and tells you what you need to charge each client in order to stay in business.

Follow the steps below to find out what is your Base Price Budget.

Step 1: Enter your information:

Line 1. Total Monthly Expense. $_____
*(enter all your **total monthly expenses**)*

Line 2. Projected Monthly Profit. $_____
*(enter the amount of profit **you want to make** Each month).*

Line 3. Total # Monthly Client Visits.   _____
*(take the # of services you have, multiply by the # of clients **each person can serve in a month**. You can use your actual client count).*

Step 2: Now calculate the information below:

Line 4: Total projected gross sales $_____
*(take the **total monthly expenses** (line 1) and Add to the **projected monthly profit** (line 2).*

Line 5: Recommended base price
*(take the total projected gross sales (line 4) $_____
And divide the total # **monthly clients visits** (line 3).*

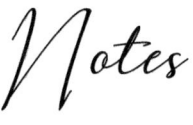

Notes

Slaying All Day!

MONDAY

WEEKEND

TUESDAY

Goals
FOR THE WEEK

WEDNESDAY

TO DO:

Task   **Done**

- [ ]
- [ ]
- [ ]
- [ ]
- [ ]
- [ ]
- [ ]
- [ ]
- [ ]
- [ ]

THURSDAY

FRIDAY

This Week's Affirmation:

Motivate your team to be a boss.

Weekly Average Ticket Tracker

Knowing your average ticket tells you what each client is spending for their services and retail products.

Step1: Enter Your Info

Line 1: Total Service Dollar $_____
(enter the weekly amt. client spent only)

Line 2: Total Retail Dollars $_____
(enter the weekly amt. client spent only)

Line 3: Total # of Clients. _____
(enter the total amt. of clients serviced per week)

Step 2: Calculate The Information:

Line 4: Your Average Ticket. $_____
(take line 1 total service dollars and divide by the total # of clients from line 3).

Line 5: Your Average Retail Ticket $_____
(take line 2 your total retail dollars and divide by the total # of clients from line 3).

Base Price Budget Worksheet

Knowing your base price calculation will help you to structure your prices for your business and tells you what you need to charge each client in order to stay in business.

Follow the steps below to find out what is your Base Price Budget.

Step 1: Enter your information:

Line 1. Total Monthly Expense. $_____
*(enter all your **total monthly expenses**)*

Line 2. Projected Monthly Profit. $_____
*(enter the amount of profit **you want to make** Each month).*

Line 3. Total # Monthly Client Visits.   _____
*(take the # of services you have, multiply by the # of clients **each person can serve in a month**. You can use your actual client count).*

Step 2: Now calculate the information below:

Line 4: Total projected gross sales $_____
*(take the **total monthly expenses** (line 1) and Add to the **projected monthly profit** (line 2).*

Line 5: Recommended base price
*(take the total projected gross sales (line 4) $_____ And divide the total # **monthly clients visits** (line 3).*

Notes

Slaying All Day!

DATE

__ __ / __ __ / __ __

MONDAY

WEEKEND

TUESDAY

Goals
FOR THE WEEK

WEDNESDAY

TO DO:

Task	Done
	☐
	☐
	☐
	☐
	☐
	☐
	☐
	☐
	☐

THURSDAY

FRIDAY

This Week's Affirmation.

Create customized experiences.

Weekly Average Ticket Tracker

Knowing your average ticket tells you what each client is spending for their services and retail products.

Step1: Enter Your Info

Line 1: Total Service Dollar $_____
(enter the weekly amt. client spent only)

Line 2: Total Retail Dollars $_____
(enter the weekly amt. client spent only)

Line 3: Total # of Clients. _____
(enter the total amt. of clients serviced per week)

Step 2: Calculate The Information:

Line 4: Your Average Ticket. $_____
(take line 1 total service dollars and divide by the total # of clients from line 3).

Line 5: Your Average Retail Ticket $_____
(take line 2 your total retail dollars and divide by the total # of clients from line 3).

Base Price Budget Worksheet

Knowing your base price calculation will help you to structure your prices for your business and tells you what you need to charge each client in order to stay in business.

Follow the steps below to find out what is your Base Price Budget.

Step 1: Enter your information:

Line 1. Total Monthly Expense. $_____
*(enter all your **total monthly expenses**)*

Line 2. Projected Monthly Profit. $_____
*(enter the amount of profit **you want to make** Each month).*

Line 3. Total # Monthly Client Visits. _____
*(take the # of services you have, multiply by the # of clients **each person can serve in a month**. You can use your actual client count).*

Step 2: Now calculate the information below:

Line 4: Total projected gross sales $_____
*(take the **total monthly expenses** (line 1) and Add to the **projected monthly profit** (line 2).*

Line 5: Recommended base price
*(take the total projected gross sales (line 4) $_____ And divide the total # **monthly clients visits** (line 3).*

Notes

Slaying All Day!

MONDAY

WEEKEND

TUESDAY

Goals
FOR THE WEEK

WEDNESDAY

TO DO:

Task	Done
	☐
	☐
	☐
	☐
	☐
	☐
	☐
	☐
	☐
	☐

THURSDAY

FRIDAY

This Week's Affirmation:

Use problems as learning experiences.

Weekly Average Ticket Tracker

Knowing your average ticket tells you what each client is spending for their services and retail products.

Step1: Enter Your Info

Line 1: Total Service Dollar $_____
(enter the weekly amt. client spent only)

Line 2: Total Retail Dollars $_____
(enter the weekly amt. client spent only)

Line 3: Total # of Clients. _____
(enter the total amt. of clients serviced per week)

Step 2: Calculate The Information:

Line 4: Your Average Ticket. $_____
(take line 1 total service dollars and divide by the total # of clients from line 3).

Line 5: Your Average Retail Ticket $_____
(take line 2 your total retail dollars and divide by the total # of clients from line 3).

Base Price Budget Worksheet

Knowing your base price calculation will help you to structure your prices for your business and tells you what you need to charge each client in order to stay in business.

Follow the steps below to find out what is your Base Price Budget.

Step 1: Enter your information:

Line 1. Total Monthly Expense. $_____
*(enter all your **total monthly expenses**)*

Line 2. Projected Monthly Profit. $_____
*(enter the amount of profit **you want to make**
Each month).*

Line 3. Total # Monthly Client Visits.   _____
*(take the # of services you have, multiply by the
# of clients **each person can serve in a month**.
You can use your actual client count).*

Step 2: Now calculate the information below:

Line 4: Total projected gross sales $_____
*(take the **total monthly expenses** (line 1) and
Add to the **projected monthly profit** (line 2).*

Line 5: Recommended base price
(take the total projected gross sales (line 4) $_____
*And divide the total # **monthly clients visits**
(line 3).*

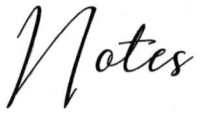

Notes

Slaying All Day!

MONDAY

WEEKEND

TUESDAY

Goals FOR THE WEEK

WEDNESDAY

THURSDAY

TO DO:

Task	Done
	☐
	☐
	☐
	☐
	☐
	☐
	☐
	☐
	☐

FRIDAY

This Week's Affirmation:

Encourage yourself in the Lord.

Weekly Average Ticket Tracker

Knowing your average ticket tells you what each client is spending for their services and retail products.

Step1: Enter Your Info

Line 1: Total Service Dollar $________________
(enter the weekly amt. client spent only)

Line 2: Total Retail Dollars $________________
(enter the weekly amt. client spent only)

Line 3: Total # of Clients. ___________________
(enter the total amt. of clients serviced per week)

Step 2: Calculate The Information:

Line 4: Your Average Ticket. $________________
(take line 1 total service dollars and divide by the total # of clients from line 3).

Line 5: Your Average Retail Ticket $_____________
(take line 2 your total retail dollars and divide by the total # of clients from line 3).

Base Price Budget Worksheet

Knowing your base price calculation will help you to structure your prices for your business and tells you what you need to charge each client in order to stay in business.

Follow the steps below to find out what is your Base Price Budget.

Step 1: Enter your information:

Line 1. Total Monthly Expense. $_____
*(enter all your **total monthly expenses**)*

Line 2. Projected Monthly Profit. $_____
*(enter the amount of profit **you want to make** Each month).*

Line 3. Total # Monthly Client Visits.   _____
*(take the # of services you have, multiply by the # of clients **each person can serve in a month**. You can use your actual client count).*

Step 2: Now calculate the information below:

Line 4: Total projected gross sales $_____
*(take the **total monthly expenses** (line 1) and Add to the **projected monthly profit** (line 2).*

Line 5: Recommended base price
*(take the total projected gross sales (line 4) $_____ And divide the total # **monthly clients visits** (line 3).*

Notes

Slaying All Day!

MONDAY

WEEKEND

TUESDAY

Goals
FOR THE WEEK

WEDNESDAY

THURSDAY

TO DO:

Task	Done
	☐
	☐
	☐
	☐
	☐
	☐
	☐
	☐
	☐

FRIDAY

This Week's Affirmation:

Don't take No for an answer.

Weekly Average Ticket Tracker

Knowing your average ticket tells you what each client is spending for their services and retail products.

Step1: Enter Your Info

Line 1: Total Service Dollar $_____
(enter the weekly amt. client spent only)

Line 2: Total Retail Dollars $_____
(enter the weekly amt. client spent only)

Line 3: Total # of Clients. _____
(enter the total amt. of clients serviced per week)

Step 2: Calculate The Information:

Line 4: Your Average Ticket. $_____
(take line 1 total service dollars and divide by the total # of clients from line 3).

Line 5: Your Average Retail Ticket $_____
(take line 2 your total retail dollars and divide by the total # of clients from line 3).

Base Price Budget Worksheet

Knowing your base price calculation will help you to structure your prices for your business and tells you what you need to charge each client in order to stay in business.

Follow the steps below to find out what is your Base Price Budget.

Step 1: Enter your information:

Line 1. Total Monthly Expense. $_____
*(enter all your **total monthly expenses**)*

Line 2. Projected Monthly Profit. $_____
*(enter the amount of profit **you want to make** Each month).*

Line 3. Total # Monthly Client Visits.   _____
*(take the # of services you have, multiply by the # of clients **each person can serve in a month**. You can use your actual client count).*

Step 2: Now calculate the information below:

Line 4: Total projected gross sales $_____
*(take the **total monthly expenses** (line 1) and Add to the **projected monthly profit** (line 2).*

Line 5: Recommended base price
(take the total projected gross sales (line 4) $_____
*And divide the total # **monthly clients visits** (line 3).*

Notes

Slaying All Day!

MONDAY

WEEKEND

TUESDAY

Goals
FOR THE WEEK

WEDNESDAY

THURSDAY

TO DO:

Task	Done
	☐
	☐
	☐
	☐
	☐
	☐
	☐
	☐

FRIDAY

This Week's Affirmation:

Prep the night before for the next day.

Weekly Average Ticket Tracker

Knowing your average ticket tells you what each client is spending for their services and retail products.

Step1: Enter Your Info

Line 1: Total Service Dollar $_____
(enter the weekly amt. client spent only)

Line 2: Total Retail Dollars $_____
(enter the weekly amt. client spent only)

Line 3: Total # of Clients. _____
(enter the total amt. of clients serviced per week)

Step 2: Calculate The Information:

Line 4: Your Average Ticket. $_____
(take line 1 total service dollars and divide by the total # of clients from line 3).

Line 5: Your Average Retail Ticket $_____
(take line 2 your total retail dollars and divide by the total # of clients from line 3).

Base Price Budget Worksheet

Knowing your base price calculation will help you to structure your prices for your business and tells you what you need to charge each client in order to stay in business.

Follow the steps below to find out what is your Base Price Budget.

Step 1: Enter your information:

Line 1. Total Monthly Expense. $_____
(enter all your **total monthly expenses**)

Line 2. Projected Monthly Profit. $_____
(enter the amount of profit **you want to make** Each month).

Line 3. Total # Monthly Client Visits. _____
(take the # of services you have, multiply by the # of clients **each person can serve in a month**. You can use your actual client count).

Step 2: Now calculate the information below:

Line 4: Total projected gross sales $_____
(take the **total monthly expenses** (line 1) and Add to the **projected monthly profit** (line 2).

Line 5: Recommended base price
(take the total projected gross sales (line 4) $_____ And divide the total # **monthly clients visits** (line 3).

Notes

Slaying All Day!

DATE
__ / __ / __

MONDAY

TUESDAY

WEDNESDAY

THURSDAY

FRIDAY

WEEKEND

Goals
FOR THE WEEK

TO DO:

Task	Done
	☐
	☐
	☐
	☐
	☐
	☐
	☐
	☐
	☐

This Week's Affirmation:

Stay focus and block out distractions.

Weekly Average Ticket Tracker

Knowing your average ticket tells you what each client is spending for their services and retail products.

Step1: Enter Your Info

Line 1: Total Service Dollar $_____
(enter the weekly amt. client spent only)

Line 2: Total Retail Dollars $_____
(enter the weekly amt. client spent only)

Line 3: Total # of Clients. _____
(enter the total amt. of clients serviced per week)

Step 2: Calculate The Information:

Line 4: Your Average Ticket. $_____
(take line 1 total service dollars and divide by the total # of clients from line 3).

Line 5: Your Average Retail Ticket $_____
(take line 2 your total retail dollars and divide by the total # of clients from line 3).

Base Price Budget Worksheet

Knowing your base price calculation will help you to structure your prices for your business and tells you what you need to charge each client in order to stay in business.

Follow the steps below to find out what is your Base Price Budget.

Step 1: Enter your information:

Line 1. Total Monthly Expense. $_____
*(enter all your **total monthly expenses**)*

Line 2. Projected Monthly Profit. $_____
*(enter the amount of profit **you want to make** Each month).*

Line 3. Total # Monthly Client Visits.   _____
*(take the # of services you have, multiply by the # of clients **each person can serve in a month**. You can use your actual client count).*

Step 2: Now calculate the information below:

Line 4: Total projected gross sales $_____
*(take the **total monthly expenses** (line 1) and Add to the **projected monthly profit** (line 2).*

Line 5: Recommended base price
(take the total projected gross sales (line 4) $_____
*And divide the total # **monthly clients visits** (line 3).*

Notes

Slaying All Day!

DATE
__ / __ / __

MONDAY

WEEKEND

TUESDAY

Goals
FOR THE WEEK

WEDNESDAY

TO DO:

Task	Done
	☐
	☐
	☐
	☐
	☐
	☐
	☐
	☐
	☐
	☐

THURSDAY

FRIDAY

This Week's Affirmation:

Take time to unwind from your day.

Weekly Average Ticket Tracker

Knowing your average ticket tells you what each client is spending for their services and retail products.

Step1: Enter Your Info

Line 1: Total Service Dollar $_____
(enter the weekly amt. client spent only)

Line 2: Total Retail Dollars $_____
(enter the weekly amt. client spent only)

Line 3: Total # of Clients. _____
(enter the total amt. of clients serviced per week)

Step 2: Calculate The Information:

Line 4: Your Average Ticket. $_____
(take line 1 total service dollars and divide by the total # of clients from line 3).

Line 5: Your Average Retail Ticket $_____
(take line 2 your total retail dollars and divide by the total # of clients from line 3).

Base Price Budget Worksheet

Knowing your base price calculation will help you to structure your prices for your business and tells you what you need to charge each client in order to stay in business.

Follow the steps below to find out what is your Base Price Budget.

Step 1: Enter your information:

Line 1. Total Monthly Expense. $_____
*(enter all your **total monthly expenses**)*

Line 2. Projected Monthly Profit. $_____
*(enter the amount of profit **you want to make** Each month).*

Line 3. Total # Monthly Client Visits.   _____
*(take the # of services you have, multiply by the # of clients **each person can serve in a month**. You can use your actual client count).*

Step 2: Now calculate the information below:

Line 4: Total projected gross sales $_____
*(take the **total monthly expenses** (line 1) and Add to the **projected monthly profit** (line 2).*

Line 5: Recommended base price
(take the total projected gross sales (line 4) $_____
*And divide the total # **monthly clients visits** (line 3).*

Notes

Slaying All Day!

MONDAY

WEEKEND

TUESDAY

Goals FOR THE WEEK

WEDNESDAY

THURSDAY

TO DO:

Task	Done
	☐
	☐
	☐
	☐
	☐
	☐
	☐
	☐
	☐
	☐

FRIDAY

This Week's Affirmation:

Evaluate what worked and what didn't then adjust.

Weekly Average Ticket Tracker

Knowing your average ticket tells you what each client is spending for their services and retail products.

Step1: Enter Your Info

Line 1: Total Service Dollar $_____
(enter the weekly amt. client spent only)

Line 2: Total Retail Dollars $_____
(enter the weekly amt. client spent only)

Line 3: Total # of Clients. _____
(enter the total amt. of clients serviced per week)

Step 2: Calculate The Information:

Line 4: Your Average Ticket. $_____
(take line 1 total service dollars and divide by the total # of clients from line 3).

Line 5: Your Average Retail Ticket $_____
(take line 2 your total retail dollars and divide by the total # of clients from line 3).

Base Price Budget Worksheet

Knowing your base price calculation will help you to structure your prices for your business and tells you what you need to charge each client in order to stay in business.

Follow the steps below to find out what is your Base Price Budget.

Step 1: Enter your information:

Line 1. Total Monthly Expense. $_____
*(enter all your **total monthly expenses**)*

Line 2. Projected Monthly Profit. $_____
*(enter the amount of profit **you want to make** Each month).*

Line 3. Total # Monthly Client Visits.   _____
*(take the # of services you have, multiply by the # of clients **each person can serve in a month**. You can use your actual client count).*

Step 2: Now calculate the information below:

Line 4: Total projected gross sales $_____
*(take the **total monthly expenses** (line 1) and Add to the **projected monthly profit** (line 2).*

Line 5: Recommended base price
(take the total projected gross sales (line 4) $_____
*And divide the total # **monthly clients visits** (line 3).*

Notes

Slaying All Day!

MONDAY

WEEKEND

TUESDAY

Goals
FOR THE WEEK

WEDNESDAY

TO DO:

Task	Done
	☐
	☐
	☐
	☐
	☐
	☐
	☐
	☐
	☐
	☐

THURSDAY

FRIDAY

This Week's Affirmation:

Declutter mentally and physically on a regular basis.

Weekly Average Ticket Tracker

Knowing your average ticket tells you what each client is spending for their services and retail products.

Step1: Enter Your Info

Line 1: Total Service Dollar $_____
(enter the weekly amt. client spent only)

Line 2: Total Retail Dollars $_____
(enter the weekly amt. client spent only)

Line 3: Total # of Clients. _____
(enter the total amt. of clients serviced per week)

Step 2: Calculate The Information:

Line 4: Your Average Ticket. $_____
(take line 1 total service dollars and divide by the total # of clients from line 3).

Line 5: Your Average Retail Ticket $_____
(take line 2 your total retail dollars and divide by the total # of clients from line 3).

Base Price Budget Worksheet

Knowing your base price calculation will help you to structure your prices for your business and tells you what you need to charge each client in order to stay in business.

Follow the steps below to find out what is your Base Price Budget.

Step 1: Enter your information:

Line 1. Total Monthly Expense. $_____
*(enter all your **total monthly expenses**)*

Line 2. Projected Monthly Profit. $_____
*(enter the amount of profit **you want to make**
Each month).*

Line 3. Total # Monthly Client Visits.   _____
*(take the # of services you have, multiply by the
# of clients **each person can serve in a month**.
You can use your actual client count).*

Step 2: Now calculate the information below:

Line 4: Total projected gross sales $_____
*(take the **total monthly expenses** (line 1) and
Add to the **projected monthly profit** (line 2).*

Line 5: Recommended base price
(take the total projected gross sales (line 4) $_____
*And divide the total # **monthly clients visits**
(line 3).*

Notes

Slaying All Day!

MONDAY

WEEKEND

TUESDAY

Goals
FOR THE WEEK

WEDNESDAY

THURSDAY

TO DO:

Task	Done
	☐
	☐
	☐
	☐
	☐
	☐
	☐
	☐
	☐

FRIDAY

This Week's Affirmation:

You can do all things through Christ.

Weekly Average Ticket Tracker

Knowing your average ticket tells you what each client is spending for their services and retail products.

Step1: Enter Your Info

Line 1: Total Service Dollar $_____
(enter the weekly amt. client spent only)

Line 2: Total Retail Dollars $_____
(enter the weekly amt. client spent only)

Line 3: Total # of Clients. _____
(enter the total amt. of clients serviced per week)

Step 2: Calculate The Information:

Line 4: Your Average Ticket. $_____
(take line 1 total service dollars and divide by the total # of clients from line 3).

Line 5: Your Average Retail Ticket $_____
(take line 2 your total retail dollars and divide by the total # of clients from line 3).

Base Price Budget Worksheet

Knowing your base price calculation will help you to structure your prices for your business and tells you what you need to charge each client in order to stay in business.

Follow the steps below to find out what is your Base Price Budget.

Step 1: Enter your information:

Line 1. Total Monthly Expense. $_____
*(enter all your **total monthly expenses**)*

Line 2. Projected Monthly Profit. $_____
*(enter the amount of profit **you want to make** Each month).*

Line 3. Total # Monthly Client Visits.   _____
*(take the # of services you have, multiply by the # of clients **each person can serve in a month**. You can use your actual client count).*

Step 2: Now calculate the information below:

Line 4: Total projected gross sales $_____
*(take the **total monthly expenses** (line 1) and Add to the **projected monthly profit** (line 2).*

Line 5: Recommended base price
(take the total projected gross sales (line 4) $_____
*And divide the total # **monthly clients visits** (line 3).*

Notes